Blooming Through the Night

Eveling Queirolo

Dedication

"To my beloved parents, Lucy and Oscar, whose unwavering love and support have been the foundation of my strength. To my sisters Jaqui, Caty, and Joyceling, my pillars of resilience and companions in every chapter of life.

To my husband James, whose unconditional love has been a constant source of comfort and inspiration. To my daughters Camila and Natalia, the lights of my life, who bring joy and purpose to every moment.

To my cherished family, friends, and colleagues, your presence and encouragement have been a guiding light through the challenges and triumphs.

To the dedicated members of my medical team, especially Dr. Saleem, your expertise, compassion, and unwavering commitment transformed the path of my breast cancer journey. This book is dedicated to each of you, with profound gratitude for being my anchors in the storm and my companions in the journey. Your love has shaped the pages of this story and enriched every chapter."

Acknowledgment

Writing this book has been a journey of reflection, healing and growth, and it would not have been possible without the support and encouragement of many incredible individuals.

First and foremost, I want to express my deepest gratitude to my husband, James.

Your unwavering love and support have been my rock, and I could not have navigated this journey without you by my side. To my two beautiful daughters, thank you for being my source of joy and inspiration every single day.

To my parents and sisters, your constant love and encouragement have given me the strength to persevere. Thank you for always believing in me and for the countless ways you have supported me. To my family and friends, thank you for your prayers, kind words, and acts of kindness. Your support has meant the world to me and has lifted me up during the toughest times. A special thank you to my medical team, who provided exceptional care and comfort. Your expertise, compassion, and encouragement have made all the difference in my journey of recovery.

To my colleagues, thank you for your understanding, flexibility, and support. Your positive energy and kindness have been a source of strength.

To my fellow cancer survivors and the breast cancer community, thank you for sharing your stories, strength, and hope.

You have shown me that we are never alone in this journey, and your courage continues to inspire me.

Finally, to every reader who picks up this book, thank you for allowing me to share my story with you. I hope my journey offers you comfort, hope, and the reminder that even in the darkest of nights, we can bloom.

With heartfelt gratitude,

Eveling Queirolo

About the Author

Eveling Queirolo is an inspiring voice, sharing her journey with strength and grace.

Originally from Peru, she brings a rich cultural perspective to her writing. Now residing in Maryland, she balances her life as a dedicated wife and mother of two daughters with her career in retail.

Her love for books, plants, travel, and decoration infuses her world with beauty, adventure, and creativity. Whether tending her garden, curating her personal library, or transforming her home into a haven, while her love for travel fuels her sense of curiosity about the world, she finds joy in the simple, meaningful moments of life. In "Blooming Through the Night", Eveling Queirolo shares her personal story of resilience and hope, offering readers a heartfelt narrative of overcoming adversity and finding light in the darkest times.

Contents

Chapter 1: Whispers of Change - Life Before Diagnosis

I am Eveling Queirolo, just as I'm not originally from the USA, so it wasn't the cancer in my breast. I find my roots in Peru, my birthplace, together with my family, and moved to the United States in 1993. I was thirteen years old when my parents decided to migrate in search of a better lifestyle and a promising future for their upcoming generations. Like any other resident from a middle-income country, my parents looked forward to a life in the developed world, where opportunities bloomed in every corner. Henceforth, together with me and my younger sisters, they took the big leap of faith.

Perceptibly, all that glitters is not gold. Our family encountered new types of hardships as we moved to the States. Livelihood was the foremost concern that hit us, and as my parents did not speak English, they had to take up lower-paying jobs upon our arrival in the new country—jobs they had never done before. My mother took up the role of cleaning houses whilst my father was hired at a restaurant to wash the dishes. As both were working two full-time jobs, and I was the next eldest person in the family, the responsibility of my younger sisters rested upon my young teenage shoulders.

It was as if the financial problems were not enough, and soon, we would have to deal with the cultural differences as well. Not being from here, my parents were not well-versed in English. This made it difficult for them to carry out their day-to-day activities like helping with our school homework, paying the bills over the phone, writing checks, attending parent conferences, etc. Consequently, that meant additional errands for me. Even if they could manage to get past the language barrier, their prolonged working hours would not have permitted them to fulfill these tasks.

Owing to all these parental duties that fate had put upon me, I matured at a young age. From the tender age of 13, I had begun to learn multi-tasking and being responsible for various decision-making responsibilities. As much as I loathed being the mother I never signed up for back in the day, I can now see that it was for the better. Little did I know that striving to be the best possible role model for my little sisters was a divine hint for preparing me for the struggles awaiting me.

Often, I found myself blaming this country for stealing away my childhood from me at a young age, forcing me to mature sooner than I was supposed to. My belief in the fact that everything happens for a reason solidified as I realized with time that had I not gone through that toilsome phase in my early life, I could never have been prepared for the bigger troubles I was bound to encounter in my later life.

I had always been a smart child at school and showed my artistic side through dancing for school in the Pom Pom dance team at Seneca Valley High School, and the Peruvian

Folk Dance "Puro Peru" group created by my Aunt Nora and Uncle Felipe kept me very busy as a teenager and young adult. As an immigrant, my family and I were fighting multiple fronts at the same time. Luckily, despite the cultural challenges, I was able to secure good grades in school. Eventually, the trend carried forward to college, where I became the first person from my family of immigrants to graduate college in the USA. It was a proud moment for all of us as I received my bachelor's degree in business with a specialization in International Business from the University of Maryland Robert H. Smith School of Business. For that, I was grateful to my parents for their laborious efforts that helped me reach there. Scrutinizing their laborious efforts from an early age made me passionate about changing the dynamics. I really wanted to give them the life they deserved and dreamt of when departing Peru. Their reliance on me kept me motivated throughout my academic and professional journey. It made me resilient enough to never give up in the worst moments. To this day, I believe it's their collective strength that keeps me going even in the face of difficulties.

Soon after graduation, I started my journey in a retail company. Owing to the remarkable environment and appreciative employers who were successful in retaining me up until now, i.e., after 19+ years. I served in several departments during my tenure here, making me an all-rounder with multi-faceted experience. Simultaneously, the consistency and reliability I showcased over the years have made me an asset to the company.

While my career advanced in full swing, my personal life could not stay behind. I found a caring and understanding man who I now proudly call my husband. After getting to know him better, we decided to start a family. I had two beautiful baby girls with him. The motherly instincts that I developed as a caretaker for my sisters came in handy while bringing them up.

As I look back, I see that that phase of my life is associated with many pleasant memories. It was the prime years of my life with a well-set career, a loving husband, two kids, a caring family, and great friends. It was picture-perfect. These blissful years were short-lived, however, as my younger daughter was diagnosed with autism. The news came as a shock to both my husband and me.

I may have only fleetingly heard the name of the neurological and developmental disorder in some social media or awareness campaigns. Therefore, I was entirely clueless about the nature of the disease and, consequently, had little knowledge of the measures to be taken in order to combat it. My husband, too, did not have sufficient medical expertise to bring him on the same page as me.

To make matters worse, she was completely non-verbal. This made it even more difficult for us to decipher her needs at the correct moment. It was an extremely challenging time for our family, especially for me and my husband. I attribute it to our teamwork, love, and understanding that prompted us to go through that rough patch in our lives.

As if being an immigrant, dealing with cultural differences, taking up mature roles at a young age, and having a daughter with special needs were enough challenges, we soon got another unpleasant news. Around my mid-thirties, my husband was diagnosed with a debilitating disease: Multiple Sclerosis. It is a neurological condition that hampers the functionality of the brain and spinal cord, gradually resulting in mild loss of functions. It hadn't been long before the worrisome news of his weakening health had been disclosed that my own health had started deteriorating. Caught up with my family's issues, I completely ignored the omens. I was 40 when suddenly, my body started undergoing inexplicable changes. It started with my left breast developing a rusty-brown patch, which would bleed every morning when I woke up.

The first few times, I found it to be something extremely unusual and unheard of. It did not hurt or appear lumpy enough to ring any bells, and thus, I kept ignoring it, hoping it would be gone by itself in a few days. Being a lady who's vigilant about her health, I regularly got my annual check-ups done with the gynecologist and primary doctor. A few months before these patches appeared, I had my last check-up, where the gynecologist did not point towards anything remotely abnormal.

As it became a routine, I decided to consult my mother as she was the closest elderly woman, or perhaps it was just an innate reflex to call *mom*. The reason I called her was not that the occurrence worried me but because it was becoming an annoying hindrance to my usual, already occupied routine.

Much to my expectations, she did not point toward anything serious either and told me that it might be due to the hormonal changes my body must be going through since I had entered the premenopausal age bracket. She further shared a similar experience she had around that age. Even if I had an ounce of doubt in me, it was completely gone after my conversations with her, and I disregarded my blood-oozing breast. I satisfied myself with the plan to discuss the occurrence with my gynecologist in our next annual appointment.

Another strange incident took place sometime later when my ability to hear things got so disrupted. I could not tell what someone was speaking unless I correlated their lips' patterns to their faint voice. It's akin to how your ears feel at the time of the take-off in a plane.

It was an extremely unsettling feeling on the brink of irritability. This was the time during the COVID-19 pandemic, and all official correspondence took place online. Zoom was the common medium for communication, and it became extremely difficult for me to comprehend what the other party was saying. When the condition did not improve in a few days, I decided to visit the doctor regarding my hearing issue as it was greatly compromising both my personal and professional lives. Meeting him was another milestone in my life, which reinforced my belief that everything happens for a reason. I began telling him about my hearing condition, complaining about how it was troubling me at work. I told him that it was not sinus, but nevertheless, he gave me medicine for its treatment.

However, even after assessing me and prescribing the medicine, the doctor wasn't satisfied. Over and over again, he kept inquiring about the reason behind my arrival here. Just like his questions, my answer was consistent. He, however, was adamant about getting to the bottom of it and prompted me to think if there was any other issue worth discussing. By this time, I had grown accustomed to the seeping breast and had almost forgotten about it. Had he not been so determined, I would have probably never mentioned it.

Upon his insistence, I gave in and told him about the brownish fluid that had been discharging from my breast for the past three months. His response to it was nothing like I had imagined; his expressions changed, and a perturbed look washed over him. He looked at me unbelievingly and questioned why I hadn't mentioned this before. I told him that this wasn't something I was there for.

As a matter of urgency, he directed me to get a mammogram done and got me the earliest appointment scheduled out of concern. At the time, his actions made little sense to me, as the most I was expecting was a blood test. But I'm forever grateful to his instincts and him as the results of the mammogram changed my life like never before!

Chapter 2: A Single Word - The Impact of Diagnosis

It was a pleasant morning; the typical Washington DC light blue sky peppered with clouds as it usually was in summer. I had just finished my chores. Everything seemed to be as normal as it could be; we were taking it for granted, clueless that from this day onwards, our lives would take a sharp turn. My husband sipped his coffee while taking our dog Coco for a walk. I was about to head out, leaving earlier than my usual time today.

I drove on a different route today as I was not going to the office, which is something that annoyed me a tad bit since it was not part of my routine. Instead, I was heading to get the mammogram done that my doctor had been so insistent upon. I had informed my boss priorly that I would be running late as I had a doctor's appointment. I didn't feel the need to tell him the details as I didn't realize it was that important of a test.

I still did not feel the need to have it done, and had he not been my doctor for several years or been so insistent, I probably would have skipped it altogether. After all, I had just turned 40 last month, so I was bound to have hormonal imbalances.

My mother had similar issues when she was my age, and I reckon most women experience such changes in their bodies as a result of menopause and other aging factors. What was it that made me stand out? I wasn't aware at that time. On top of that, I always took good care of my feminine health. I always attended the yearly checkups with my gynecologist. I even did monthly checkups and often palpated my breasts in case of the occurrence of some lump. Why couldn't a simple blood test point out the issue, I wondered. Nevertheless, I will be having my follow-up checkup with my gynecologist by the end of the year. What was the point of this urgency? The more I thought about it, the more irritation I felt towards my doctor. Nonetheless, his knowledge and experience precede mine and the women around me, so trusting him was the wisest thing to do.

I had never had a mammogram done before and wondered what it might feel like. Is there a protocol that I would have to follow inside? Would it be painful? Is there something I was supposed to prepare prior that I was unaware of a new train of thoughts that had now taken over my mind?

After driving for about twenty-five minutes, I reached the place. It was a small but well-maintained place, and the healthcare staff were wearing their usual white, green, and blue garments, depending on their role. A nurse clad in white took me to a room where they were supposed to carry out the test. The door had a label hinged to it that warned of radioactivity. That day, I learned that mammograms are simply low-grade X-rays. They took me to this machine, around nine feet tall, with a small tray in the middle. The protocol was to place the breast on it. The height of the tray was adjusted for me as I did how the nurse instructed. Another parallel plate from the top squeezed my breast to keep it in place. It was done from multiple sides to get a view from different angles.

Every time she squeezed them to get a shot, a lot of blood mixed with other fluids discharged from my breast. I wasn't quite alarmed as it has been going on for months since I started having this discharge. It was much more blood than usual, so much so that the whole table was covered in blood. However, I thought it was probably because she was squeezing it too hard. This was one of the red flags I had missed. The other red flag I missed was the nurse frantically coming and going, performing more and more tests every time.

After a while, she returned and told me that they needed to run a breast ultrasound and that I'd need to move to a different room. I didn't mind changing rooms, but I wondered what it was like with so many tests. Now I had started to get worried, remembering the expression on my doctor's face when I told him about the condition of my breast, him prescribing a mammogram, the nurse going to and from, and now another test. It all added up to an impending bad news.

Even in this state of anguish, the most I could think about was the doctor coming up at the end of it all and giving me some high dose of medicine to control the chaotic hormones. Not even in my worst dreams could I have imagined what I was told. In the ultrasound room, there was another nurse who catered to me. She was called the sonographer as she specialized in those scans. As I lay there, she placed the probe on my breast and took pictures from the screen in front of her. The room was dreadfully quiet. She never spoke throughout the process, and neither did I. The only noise in the room was the humming of the machine and the faint static of the electric cables.

After collecting sufficient information, she went outside only to shortly return with a lady in navy blue scrubs, who I presumed to be the doctor. She, too, maintained the quiet of the room as she proceeded to take more pictures without the exchange of a single word. It looked like she was trying to verify the findings of the sonographer before her. Once she was done, she sat beside me, maintaining eye level, her manner quite composed and calculated as this was something she did quite often. Without making any grounds or sugarcoating her words, she plainly uttered the words, "You have cancer zero DCIS."

I have what?

Here I was, thinking she was about to prescribe me drugs for hormonal imbalance. I was caught completely off-guard and looked at her petrified. I couldn't focus on whatever else she said as the word "cancer" cast a dark shadow on everything else that was going around. For a moment, I could not believe my ears and thought that I must have misheard something, but her staunchly piercing gaze portrayed another story.

It showed confidence in her claims, and what she said was as true as my existence. Nevertheless, I was in utter shock as my mind was not able to process what she had just revealed to me. I did not know or did not have the forte in me to muster a reaction. Again, she broke the silence by asking if I had any questions. Yes, there were many, but I just didn't know how to put them into words. I was still struggling with registering the news. I knew even if I tried to ask anything, the words wouldn't naturally pour out. I meekly said no, unable to utter another word. It felt as if someone had stabbed my back out of nowhere, leaving me flabbergasted. She told me she was willing to discuss it in the upcoming days once I had recollected myself. Was I ever going to recover from this news?

I waited until I was alone to pour out my sentiment. I went into the changing room to change back into my clothes, as I had been draped in a bathrobe for convenience while running the test. I burst into hysterical crying. This had been my first normal reaction ever since I got the nerve-wracking news. I cried and cried for what felt like hours without a pause. My world seemed to be shifting at an unprecedented rate as I didn't know what to think. Eventually, I caught control of my feelings, or rather tears, because emotionally, I was still all over the place. I wiped my face and went out as if nothing had happened. At the counter, I asked if I owed any payments, to which they told me I didn't. Thus, I exited the place and went to my car in the parking lot.

This was where the second fit of crying consumed me as I started rolling again. I was in desperate need of a human presence, so I quickly called my husband. At the time, he was driving and put on speaker somewhere with one of our daughters, which is something I completely ignored as I was not in my right mind and wasn't thinking straight. When he asked me about how the appointment went, I uncontrollably just blurted out the news to him. At that time, I didn't realize this was very strong news for a child, and I should have thought my words through. But at that moment, I don't think my mind was operating as usual. I couldn't imagine how he must have taken the news as he, too, was expecting it to be just another regular exam. There was silence on the other end of the phone for a few moments, followed by a panic-driven response, "What's going on? No, no, no. What are you saying?"

I knew he had heard me loud and clear but couldn't register the news, just like I couldn't when the doctor told me so. Just to be sure, I repeated myself, blabbering about what happened at the clinic, words stumbling upon one another. He tried to calm me down by saying a lot of things, but all I heard was, "Everything will be okay," and those four words have been the most soothing medicine in that tumultuous time of distress. I had now started to realize the events of the day and the calamity that had just dawned upon me. I could now recall the words of the doctor that echoed in my brain like a devilish whisper. "You have cancer, zero DCIS." It had finally started hitting me.

What exactly does it mean? Zero? Do I have cancer or not? What does DCIS stand for? Does it have a cure? Am I going to die?

A plethora of similar questions started racing through my mind.

Pushing away the bedlam in my head, I picked up my phone to call my mother and sisters. We had a group chat, so I conveniently called them. I informed them that I had cancer in the exact words that the doctor had revealed to me. After a few moments of pause, they started crying, and I joined along. I somewhat felt bad for putting my family through such difficult times, even though nothing was my fault. My younger sister went to school for medical science and was able to comprehend the technical jargon that had gone over my head. She started questioning me to make more sense of the situation. She asked me what type of cancer it was and if I could tell a bit more.

"All I understood was stage zero DCIS," I told her.

Pertinent to her profession, she replied in a composed manner, "Okay, that's good. It's not that advanced. There's a lot that you can do. There's a lot of technology. So, calm down and go home."

I asked her who I was supposed to meet and what the plan of action should be from this point forward, and she told me we needed to see an oncologist next, i.e., a cancer specialist and probably a breast surgeon. She kept prompting me to think about the next steps instead of sulking at the news, but I just couldn't keep my mind off what I had just learned and could barely focus on what she was saying. While my husband's consoling had been very emotionally comforting, having it from my sister, who was also in the medical field, had been promising. I could rely more on her words as she wasn't speaking out of mere hope but knew the technical possibilities behind it. I wiped my tears once again and began to drive back home. My teary eyes clouded the road ahead as I couldn't control myself and cried all my way home.

Coincidentally, my husband and I pulled up to our driveway at the same time. I immediately got out of my car and ran to hug him. "I have cancer," I started crying as I said those words. I gave him a big hug as my daughters joined in. I still did not realize how this news would affect their naïve minds.

At that time, my eldest daughter was only twelve, while the younger was ten only. They just hugged me and said, "Mommy, everything's going to be okay." It was at that moment that I wanted to get rid of the disease by hook or by crook. The thought of my children bothered me as they were too young to navigate life on their own and depended on me. I wondered how I'd be able to beat this deadly disease—too many unanswered questions.

The rest of the day is quite a blur in my memory. I remember lying on the sofa, just thinking and crying the whole time. My life shattered right in front of me. I just thought I was going to die. Paired with the assumption came the thought of my family, and I felt horrible leaving my kids and my husband behind. I recall questioning God. I have been a kind and helpful person who never harmed anyone.

Why is this happening to me? Where did I mess up? When did I do something wrong? Did I hurt someone? Am I being punished?

I rewound my life in search of those answers and thought until the point my head hurt, and eventually, I drifted to sleep.

In times like these, it's human nature to think of the worst-case scenarios. I could think of every pessimistic thing as possible instead of diverting my mind towards more positive and promising outcomes. In a state of hopelessness, I couldn't imagine what would happen if I could not survive and if no treatment worked on me. My kids needed me as they were too young. They were just little girls.

My husband had recently been diagnosed with multiple sclerosis and was in need of care himself. On top of that, I was the one taking care of other responsibilities at home, like paperwork and keeping track of doctors' appointments. It scared me to think of how all these duties would be managed. My relatively positive side encouraged me to stay resilient during these toilsome times. It told me that I had to fight off this disease for the sake of my family and needed to find a cure for it. I started thinking about what my sister had told me earlier.

Do I need to have surgery? Do I need to go to chemo? Do I need to get my breasts removed? Do they just extract that part that has cancer? So many questions bombarded my head, and I did not have an answer.

The next morning, I wanted to forget the events of the day before as if it had been a bad nightmare and that none of them had actually happened. But life goes on, and you can't hide away from reality. Cleaning my breast's discharge that day felt so much worse, and it reminded me of the bitter truth. I wished I had taken it more seriously.

Anyway, I proceeded with the day and went to work. Despite covering my eyes in ample amounts of concealer, the dullness in my eyes and puffiness around them gave away the state of my mind. Throughout the day, I couldn't help but cry. It was especially embarrassing when colleagues would be passing by me and see me crying, adding to the awkwardness. That day, I just wanted to hide away and not have anyone see me. I was doubting my capabilities while the questions about survival from this fatal disease kept ringing in my head. It was extremely hard for me to pretend with such questions in my mind.

A similar state of mind continued to haunt me at home as well, and I continued crying. I was not able to perform my daily tasks as efficiently as I pondered where life was taking me. I felt terrible for being the mom with cancer. I felt like I failed my babies. I may not have felt this way back then, but looking back at the time, I could tell I was extremely depressed. I was absent-minded most of the time, constantly trying to figure out what I was to do next. I scheduled appointments with multiple oncologists and breast cancer surgeons after extensively searching for the best ones in town. The logical part of me, the one I personally refer to as the project manager in me, could not stand having an uncertain future. I wanted answers and a plan of action. It had already analyzed the problem and sought ways to resolve it. This part of me helped me to keep going and hindered me from giving up or losing hope.

Through my experience, I would like all my fellow ladies going through similar dark patches in their lives to take a bold front the way I did. Remember, cancer is not stronger than you, and things will get better no matter what stage you're in. You just need to hold on and allow those survival instincts to kick in.

Chapter 3: Bearing Courage - Facing the Initial Storm

This was a race against life, and there was no time to sit and sulk. I had to reach the finish line before my cancer could reach it. Mind you, these cells multiply at lightning speed, making it exceptionally difficult for someone like me who was new to the game and completely unaware of the rules. The only rule I knew was that giving up was not an option.

For all my fellow breasties, I understand this is not an easy path, and I, strong as I probably sound now, wasn't quite like that throughout. It was an extremely difficult and unpredictable path to tread, with its own highs and lows. There were times I found immense strength and resilience, while in others, I felt weak and hopeless, as you'll see throughout this chapter. Before meeting an oncologist, I needed biopsy reports that he could use to analyze my condition and draw further plans of action. The one I was recommended was called a mammogram biopsy, which was scheduled for a week later, right after they gave me the horrifying news about cancer.

I remember that week was spent grieving as I tried to make myself believe the harsh reality that was thrown at me. My eyes were red and puffy due to constant crying. My house was in shambles, and my family was a mess; nothing seemed to matter compared to the news I was still absorbing.

A week later came the day that I will probably never forget. As it was my first experience with having a biopsy, I was entirely clueless about how it was going to be. It was the week I could have used to prepare for the procedure was spent crying in vain. Hence, I went back to the clinic, where they told me I had cancer. A feeling of anxiety and despair ran into me, and I felt scared. I was made to change into the medical robe and sit on a chair where a big needle was in front of my face.

I patiently sat there as the nurse then administered me with some local anesthesia. After a few minutes of allowing the numbness to take over, I felt a spear going deep into my breast. As the surgeon drew it deeper through my breast, I felt an excruciatingly intense pain take over. I had no clue that this was going to hurt so much.

Assuming this is how it's supposed to feel like, I kept on bearing the agonizing pain. It didn't feel like I was under the effect of anesthesia as I could profoundly feel the spear piercing inside me. Just to give you an idea about myself, I am a person with a very high pain tolerance, but this was just beyond me. Tears continuously went down my face, and I could not even feel them in lieu of my breast pain. I was not yet over the emotional pain of getting the news of cancer, and the physical hurt had begun already. I just sit there, questioning God for making me feel this way, shocked by all the pain that I was going through.

As if the pain wasn't traumatizing enough, I was losing blood with the same intensity. The amount of blood made me wonder if there was any left in me. Probably not enough, as I was drifting away in unconsciousness. Simultaneously, I had turned pale white.

This was a condition of emergency, as the staff stopped working at my breast and quickly turned me upside down and elevated my legs. Another member fetched me some orange juice. I recovered in a few minutes, and they continued piercing my breast, and the dreadfully painful experience continued. I wished there was an alternate, less painful test they could perform to get the information they needed. Two days after biopsy day — I call it biopsy day because it was a very traumatic day for me – I had an appointment scheduled with my oncologist. Just as biopsy day was full of pain, this day was full of surprises and, unfortunately, not pleasant ones.

First, as I walked in, I was the youngest person in the room, surrounded by women who seemed to be beyond their 80s. I felt so out of place, but hey, I wasn't at a party; I was at an oncologist doctor's office. The fact that we were all patients is what made us similar. Anyways, soon it was my turn, and I walked in and took my seat across the doctor. The next unprecedented thing that day was the first question he asked.

"Do you have a will?"

Do I have a what? I denied it, but the question really shocked me. *Why was he asking me that?*

It was bizarre and opened a Pandora's box of all sorts of questions and possibilities. It's human nature to picture the worst possible scenario in times of distress, and so his question made me wonder if I was going to die. It immediately worried me about my family and how they would manage without me. Eventually, I realized it was a standard oncology protocol to ask that, and as it was my first experience with one, I was unaware of it. Nevertheless, for a person who had recently found out about their cancer, this, in my opinion, was a very insensitive question to ask.

The information he had received so far was not sufficient, and hence, I was directed to get an MRI scan done. Immediately after the appointment, I went to my car and scheduled one.

MRI Scan day arrived, and it wasn't painful. However, being enclosed in a capsule for 45 minutes did make me slightly claustrophobic. This discomfort was reasonable in light of the disease, and I told myself that this was something that I had to get done. I tried to distract myself from the situation by focusing on the blissful memories I had had with my family. I reminisced about the family vacation we have had. Taking my mind off of different places that I enjoyed the most really helped calm my nerves down in that capsule.

All the pain, emotional and physical distress, and discomfort were only one aspect of the problems I was facing. Finances incurred during these procedures and appointments were an entirely different story I was faced with. MRI scans, biopsies, and doctor's appointments were quite an additional burden on the budget despite having medical insurance. This additional drain was a lot to deal with, given the emotional turmoil I was already going through.

Something I am extremely grateful for during this difficult time is the support I had from my friends and family. I always knew I had them to count upon. However, despite all their support, they couldn't really understand what I was feeling. At the end of the day, you have to bear your pain yourself, as no one else can do it for you. They were always lifting my spirits with their kind words and affirmations. However, I had to go through that process all alone. Even the most genuinely caring person could not share that pain, that far from the unknown, with me. It was this newness that really made me feel lonely down this road. I never doubted their support, but just not knowing what to expect was something that consumed me.

After I had the results of the scan and biopsy, it was time to consult the breast surgeon. This was during the Covid-19 pandemic, and thus, I had a really hard time finding a doctor. The appointment I got was after 15 days. It was kind of good, now that I look back at it, as it gave me the chance to brace myself for the next bad news. My sister, who was attending school in Florida, was visiting for the summer and accompanied me to this appointment to understand things directly in her medical jargon. I was really relieved to have her along.

After waiting for about 20 minutes, I was called into his office. We all wore masks due to the pandemic, but I could tell from his aura that he was well-versed in his field. He was tall and had dark hair. I sat across from him in order to discuss the treatment plan for the developing cancer in my left breast. It seems as if healthcare professionals secretly attend a workshop on delivering opening statements that could give horror movie jump scares a run for their money. I get it; honesty is the best policy, but maybe they could sprinkle in a little cushioning before dropping the bomb.

His version was, "So, we're here to discuss your right breast." I thought he may have confused it, so I went ahead to correct him and said, "No, we're here to talk about my left breast. DCIS, Cancer Zero...?" He frowned and looked at the papers in front of him to correct himself, but unfortunately, it was I who was indeed mistaken. He spoke with confidence, backed by the evidence in front of him that exhibited the detection of a mass in my right breast. I was stunned to learn this new piece of information and completely fell at a loss for words.

The news was such a blow that I lost track of my thoughts and the questions I had planned on asking regarding my LEFT breast. He further went on to explain that it wasn't confusing as the big white mass detected in my right breast was in place in **ADDITION TO** the mass in my left one.

When I heard those words, it immediately felt like I was very short of breath. I just couldn't comprehend what he was telling me at this point. I began tearing up like crazy, crying my heart out. All the composure I had mustered in the past fifteen days had evaporated into thin air. To be sure of it further, he also performed a manual examination, looking for lumps, but he didn't have to palpate it as the blood oozing from it was a telltale of the abnormal growth inside.

I hysterically cried on and on, shocked to hear the news. Nothing could have prepared me for this mental torture. Thankfully, my sister was there to give me the moral support I direly needed at that moment, but nothing seemed to help.

I hadn't completely taken in this news that he dropped the next bomb: in order to further analyze, he said he needed an MRI biopsy done.

AGAIN?! I thought.

The dark memories of the previous biopsy began haunting me; it was barely a month ago, and even the scars had not yet vanished completely. *How could I take another one?* I remembered how terribly painful the experience was and did not want to go through it again. The meeting with him was inundated by appalling and disconcerting news.

He told me that based on the size of the mass on my left breast, which measured six centimeters. He highly recommended a mastectomy — the complete removal of a breast. When he said that, I started to cry all over again. I was taken back as that was the first time that a doctor had told me I needed a mastectomy.

Until this point, I had been consoling myself by considering the removal through the chemical method, and I wouldn't need to lose my breast. I had been thinking that this was cancer zero and, hence, it wouldn't need any such major surgeries, but he burst my bubble in a second. It was hard to swallow the idea of losing it all. I didn't want to imagine myself without breasts; it was a horrible thought. The last nail in the coffin that day was BRCA. When he told me to get this BRCA test done, I was too mentally exhausted to solve any more medical riddles and asked what it meant. He explained that this was a gene mutation test, and since I was only 40, healthy, and with no inherited history of cancer, it was quite unusual for me to catch this disease. He further went on to explain its purpose, which was the actual news. He mentioned that if I was positive, my sisters and daughters may have a chance to have this BRCA gene as well, putting them at risk for breast cancer at some point in life.

This news left me terrified. Bearing something on yourself is one thing, but imagining it on a loved one is completely devastating. It was a bolt out of the blue. I was aware and had somewhat made peace with the fact that I had to go through a painful process in order to get rid of the disease, but never in my worst dreams could I have imagined it to overshadow my family like this. My sisters were as dear to me as my daughters, and the thought of seeing them go through all that pain was unbearable. So far, I had only gone through one procedure, and that had been gut-wrenching.

This was not where the bad news ended; he went on to explain that people with a positive BRCA have a 60-80% chance of developing ovarian cancer as well. Therefore, to avoid the possibility of it, they would need to remove both of my ovaries as well. It was a lot of information to be thrown at me at once.

I was devastated, to say the least. It seemed like every time this man spoke, bad news came out of his mouth. I didn't want to stay in his clinic anymore; I didn't have the strength in me to take any more jolts. Losing my breast and potentially my ovaries was a lot to take in. That is just the tip of the iceberg, for I had read all sorts of accounts from women who underwent menopause or the removal of their fertile organs. The aging process becomes much faster, with the skin starting to wrinkle and sag. There are hot flashes, painful back and aching knees, and a plethora of other side effects. I was too young to go through that, but there was little that could be done.

It took me two weeks to get the results of the BRCA test. Those two weeks felt like an eternity, but the wait was worth it! Two weeks later, I found that I was negative. This was the first good news in the past few months, and I was extremely relieved to know that my family was safe. These results also clarified the dread of having my ovaries removed.

Simultaneously, I had also scheduled the MRI biopsy as he recommended. However, I couldn't get it on my first visit since the location where I scheduled the appointment only had an ultrasound machine to perform the biopsy, and I needed the MRI biopsy. They did not have the designated machinery for it. It took me some time, but I didn't mind because I was learning new things daily.

During this time, I learned there are three different types of biopsies: mammogram, ultrasound, and an MRI biopsy. I rescheduled the appointment for the right biopsy. I couldn't wait for its result either, as I could only move forward with my treatment after I had its results.

It was different from the one I had had before, as this was an MRI biopsy. Before the procedure, I was extremely worried and scared, for I had been through this procedure once, and it had been excruciatingly painful. I asked the technician to administer me with some extra anesthesia, given my past experience. This surprised her, and she asked me why I wanted that.

I explained the extreme pain I felt the last time as if two spears were being pierced through me. She asked if I had told my technician about that. I hadn't, as it was my first time getting it done, and I had no idea how painful it was supposed to be. I quietly tolerated the pain, thinking it was standard protocol. Probably, the news of cancer had made me feel that way. I thought it necessary to bear that much pain, but to my surprise, this woman told me I was mistaken. "It's not supposed to hurt that bad, barely more than a pinch; you should have told your healthcare provider then only."

At that moment, I felt like such a fool. I could have saved myself from that trauma only if I had simply advocated for myself. While I was relieved that it wouldn't happen again, I felt bad that I bore it in the first place.

Therefore, for all my breasties out there, I'd like you to learn from my experience and **_DON'T MAKE ASSUMPTIONS_**. Properly do your research before any procedure and know what to expect. Even if you don't, learn to vouch for yourself. You are your biggest advocate and must stand for your health.

Based on my request, the technician agreed to give me extra anesthesia regardless. This biopsy went really well, and all I felt was a pinch when they were inserting the needle in my breast.

Once survival was in check, I spared time for the aesthetics and decided to meet a plastic surgeon as he would perform that reconstructive surgery after they removed the breast.

I learned multiple techniques for reconstructing the lost organ. Implants were to be placed under or over the muscle, using it as a support to anchor them in place. Unfortunately, however, my nipples could not be saved in any way. Initially, I would get a breast tissue expander used after a mastectomy to increase the amount of breast tissue. Once I reached the ideal size, they were to perform the final reconstructive surgery, but that is something I do not worry about at the moment. Soon after I received the results of the MRI biopsy, I got another great news, much like that of a negative BRCA. The mass in my right chest was not cancerous. It had the potential to develop into one at a later stage. The professionals gave me the option of keeping it or getting rid of it.

As you can see, a wide variety of healthcare professionals, including oncologists, breast surgeons, technicians, plastic surgeons, etc., presented me with different news each day, laying down the possible treatment plans. One day, I was just sitting with my friends and family, discussing the thoughts that had been troubling me regarding fear of surgery and loss of my natural breasts and nipples. Then, it occurred to them that I should consider taking second opinions to make more informed decisions. It wasn't a bad idea. There was a possibility that some expert might come up with a way to save my breast or suggest a better treatment option. It would give me an eagle-eye view of the situation, I thought. That is when I decided to explore more consultants and navigate my way to an efficient treatment. The cancer had waged this war against me and my loved ones. I had to make sure I won it in the best way possible.

Read on to see how I made that happen.

Chapter 4: Navigating The Maze-Understanding Treatment Options

Amidst the growing chaos, I had an intuition that I shouldn't settle with just a single diagnostic. I figured it was probably better to make a proper learned decision and get a second opinion. So, I researched online for doctors around my area and came across one of the head directors of the Breast Cancer Suburban Hospital, a very well-known medical institution.

I called to ask them about an appointment at the beginning of September, and their latest vacant spot was in late September. Based on the urgency, I just couldn't wait around that long to have a second opinion. So, I started calling other places, but there was no availability, and understandably so, since it was COVID around that time and appointments were very scarce. I had to get an appointment anyhow, so I ended up confirming my spot on the 27th of September. A week after I had booked my appointment, I was too anxious. I kept telling myself, "Oh Gosh, three weeks left until I finally get the answer on how to get rid of this cancer." I got so anxious that I couldn't wait, so I called them again to ask if there had been any cancellations and asked about the possibility of moving my appointment to a closer date.

I kept calling them on a daily basis and was very insistent. She was the director, so naturally, everyone went to her. I kept calling them, and a week later, an opening popped up for 8th September. However, this opening wasn't for the director but for her partner, Dr. Sun. My intuition kicked in, and I went and confirmed the appointment with the partner doctor. I couldn't wait three weeks. So, two days later, my appointment date with the breast surgeon finally came. I got to the doctor's office and filled out all the necessary paperwork at the reception. When the time came for me to see the doctor, I was very straightforward with her. I said, "I'm here because I want to hear a second opinion. These are my mammograms, biopsies test results, MRI CDs, etc. I want to know what other options are available and if there's anything else that could be done apart from a mastectomy."

I was really scared of it. I started praying with all my might that she would suggest something else other than a mastectomy. However, once she reviewed all my results and went through the CDs (it felt like <u>an</u> awfully long time), she finally said, "Without a doubt, you need a mastectomy. You won't be able to go very far if you don't go through with it."

So, it turned into a personal decision now. I had to decide by myself what was best for me. She continued, "As a doctor, it is my duty to tell you about all the options available. So, in regards to your right breast, you can skip it for now if you want, but it's up to you. I can only give you the facts and statistics."

The chances that I was going to get breast cancer on my right breast, based on the fact that I already had cancer, were uncertain. But, that percentage was bound to increase each year. She explained this to me and said, "Since you're only 40 years old now, you still have many years left to live. So, the risk of developing cancer in the right breast is higher in your case as the potential percentage would increase each year." I understood the message she was trying to convey, and this key information helped me make a decision.

Another news that she broke to me, which wasn't shared by my previous doctor, was that I was Hormone Receptor Negative.

This terminology was new to me at the time, but I learned that it meant I had no estrogen or progesterone receptors due to my cancer. Hence, I couldn't opt for any kind of hormonal treatment. Statistically, this type of cancer tends to grow a lot faster than a person who is Hormone Receptor Positive.

She further went over a few other things like DCIS: Ductal carcinoma in situ is the presence of abnormal cells inside a milk duct in the breast, and cancer zero means it hasn't spread outside of its original location in the breast tissue. The way she explained everything to me, including the options I had, the chances, and the numbers, made me feel very pleased and assured. The reason is that I have been a very analytical person from the start. So, for me, statistics are very important. As she went over everything, I thought, *"Finally, someone who speaks my language."* I grasped each and everything that she put forward and felt very intrigued. This led me to decide that she was the one I wanted to continue seeing. Once she was finished with her explanations, I said to her, "I will be very pleased to be your patient. What do I need to do now?" She took me in, guiding me through the whole process, where the nurse came in with a binder containing all the steps that needed to be followed. She informed me, "Since you're a Hormone Receptor Negative, the cancer will grow a lot faster. So, you need to be in the surgery room within three weeks max."

This urgency was another thing that I did not get from the previous doctor. I was beginning to feel content with my decision to get a second opinion. I thought to myself, "Thank God, I'm in the right hands now." She was the best doctor for me.

I immediately went through the paperwork to switch my doctors. When I reached there, the doctor had already contacted her plastic surgeon. She mentioned to me at some point that she had worked with this surgeon for the past ten years, so that got me a bit more reassured. My appointment with the plastic surgeon was booked for the next day at 8 am.

Ever since I learned about my cancer, for once, I felt like I was the one being taken care of. Before this, I made all the appointments by myself, tried to contact the doctors by myself, and did other things by myself. I felt like she had my back now. I felt very happy with my decision to change doctors. It was definitely the right thing to do, as she cared for me and spoke my analytical language.

So, the next day, I went to see the plastic surgeon. The meeting was fairly easy, probably the easiest one I had been to in the last three months. I told him about my diagnosis with the second doctor and how I was still indecisive if I wanted to go through with a mastectomy on my right breast or not because there was no cancer, but with the chances now being higher because of my age; I had to potentially consider it if I want to get this effectively done and over with.

The doctor calmed me down and assured me that I didn't have to make a decision right away. I had one week before surgery day to make my decision. It would then decide how many hours I would have to spend in the surgery room. The previous plastic surgeon recommended implants under the muscle. However, he explained that he preferred putting the implants over the muscle as it's less painful and takes less time for recovery.

It also looks better just in general. He had also told me about the way implants were done ten years ago. Back then, they would do it under muscle, which wasn't very efficient. He seemed like he was up-to-date with the trends. I felt fairly confident about switching between my plastic surgeon and my breast surgeon. I loved how he was on top of the new methods and made recommendations accordingly. But again, we know that there are a lot of decisions to be made while going through this whole process, and after the plastic surgeon, I had a follow-up appointment with my breast surgeon.

I had to decide if I was going to let them remove my right breast, too, or just the left one. I had one week to educate myself on the topic. I conducted thorough research, joined Facebook groups, and posted questions like, "Help, this is my situation. What decision would you guys make?" Most of the responses I received were from women who had to remove both beasts and suggested that I do, too.

I could not envision myself going through the same pain again, so I went forward with the decision to remove both of them. I, alongwith the doctors, decided it would be a Bilateral Mastectomy. I couldn't spare my left nipple because of the risk of leaving it as it was too great. Now, because the cancer had already developed in my left breast, they had to remove one of the lymph nodes in between my left arm and armpit to make sure that there wasn't any spread.These decisions were made in mid-September, and I was in constant communication with the breast surgeon coordinator to have my surgery scheduled. My surgery was finally scheduled for 6th October, my oldest and dearest niece's birthday, Jaylin.

The yin and yang was a very special day for me, but at the same time, I was about to experience a scary and painful surgery. It was scheduled in a way that aligned perfectly with everything. I had to spend some time with the breast surgeon as well as the plastic surgeon. They both wanted to make sure that the surgery was completed as soon as possible because I was a Hormone Receptor Negative, and the cancer was growing fast. I had 15 days to ensure that I had a plan in place for my work transition. I was an IT manager for a Retail store; it was the busiest time of the year.

I constantly worried that I would be letting my company down by being absent at the best time of the year, but at the same time, I also knew that if I didn't miss work now, I might not even be here by next year. I had to be a little selfish for once.

Since I was the one who took care of our house's paperwork, bills, and doctor's appointments, I made sure that my tasks for the next month were already finished. I did enough work to lighten the responsibilities that would weigh me down once I returned after a month and sat on my computer. There were a lot of things to get done in 15 days, and I had to work on the FMLA process with my company, which ensured that I would be paid despite my absence. It was too frustrating, but thankfully, I had a great support team. All my friends and family members came over days before my surgery and gave me gifts that were going to be useful during and after my surgery. My aunt,

Miluska, who owned a house cleaning company, came over and said, "My crew will come over to clean up your house while you are recovering. It's going to be a lot of work for your husband alone." My parents and sisters also showed up almost every day. I felt content as I went into surgery.As a family, Halloween was our favorite holiday, and ever since my girls were babies, we attended the pumpkin patch every year. I was heartbroken because I had surgery in 10 days, and we were all prepping up for that. I said to my husband, "I don't know if I'm going to be here for this year's pumpkin patch." On October 5th, I sent a note to my daughter's school. I told them that I would not be sending my girls to school because we were going to the Pumpkin Patch. I wanted to make sure that the tradition continued, even if I wasn't there to be a part of it. So, we did a Pumpkin Patch, and I got to spend some extra bonding time with my girls. They were very understanding and empathic to the whole situation.

Also, on the same day, I had to pay a visit to my plastic surgeon so that I could get my breasts marked. The instrument looked like a Sharpie, but it was probably just a special type of marker. It had blue ink, and I had to be marked one day before because I had to be at the hospital by five in the morning for my surgery.

Once he was done drawing, I took a picture and could see where the cuts would go and where the things would be removed. It was very intense for me because it felt like I was taking my last breath in front of a mirror and seeing all those marks. My spirit was heavy, and I cried all the way back home. I knew it was a step I must take, but I don't think I was ever ready for such an experience.

Chapter 5: Triumphs and Tribulations - The Rollercoaster of Emotions

I stared up at the ceiling, watching the faint glow of the streetlights dance across the walls as another car passed by outside. Sleep seemed determined to avoid me that night, with anxiety swirling endlessly in the dark boundaries of my mind. *What would happen once I was wheeled into that operating room? Would the surgery go as planned, or would some unforeseen complication arise? Would I make it back to my family?* Doubt and uncertainty kept dragging me back to the cold reality of what lay ahead in the morning.

When the first rays of dawn finally crept through the windows, I barely slept. My husband and I rose quietly, neither of us speaking much as we went through the motions of getting ready—the weight of what this day could bring hung heavy in the air. I kissed my kids 'goodbye,' and my parents drove my girls to their school that day. My husband came along with me to the hospital. It was a quiet ride. I cried all the way there. We arrived at the hospital far earlier than my scheduled check-in time, but to me, each minute dragged on like an hour as I waited restlessly in the pre-op area.

That's when family and friends started sending encouraging texts, wishing me well for the surgery. It was also then that my cousin Briselita happened to mention my grandfather's sister had breast cancer. Hearing that made my heart sink. *Could the disease run in my family after all?* I'd always assumed my risk was average, with no close relatives affected, but now that possibility seemed all too real.

Eventually, a nurse called me back to begin prepping for the surgery. As she took my vitals and asked routine questions, the anesthesiologist introduced himself and explained what he would do to ensure I remained unconscious and comfortable during the procedure. His calm, reassuring manner helped ease some of my nerves. Then, my plastic surgeon came by to double-check the markings drawn on my breast the previous day, making a few minor adjustments to the lines. Finally, my breast cancer surgeon spoke with me briefly as well, going over what they hoped to accomplish in the operating room.

As the surgeons explained the procedure, I focused on steadying my breathing. The radioactive tracer blue dye was injected into the skin near my breast before my surgery so they could check if the cancer had spread. Then, they needed to remove a lymph node from my left armpit. This procedure is called a sentinel lymph node biopsy. Hearing I could never have blood drawn from that arm again sent a new spike of fear through me as if I didn't have enough reminders of what I was facing. My breast surgeon spoke soothingly, seeing the panic in my eyes. He outlined each step they would take and the estimated time.

All too soon, the pre-op preparations were complete. The nurse came and told me that she was ready to take me to the operating room. I hugged my husband so hard, like it was going to be the last time, and I started to cry. As I started drifting apart from my husband, all the fears and anxiety boiled in a wave of panic.

I shook uncontrollably as they wheeled me into the bright white room. Voices sounded far away as I pleaded internally not to be left alone. The nurse gently encouraged me to think of happy memories. But nothing could still my racing thoughts. Once I arrived at the operating room, it was cold; the walls were white, and there was a bright light right above my face. As they placed the anesthetic mask over my face, my final recollection was of that blinding white light above me. Then darkness swept in, and the rest was a blank slate until slowly awakening in the recovery room. I was wrapped in bandages from chest to waist, like a mummy emerging from their wrappings.

My surgery was complete, but the recovery was only just beginning. I slept fitfully that first night, troubled by uncomfortable aches and pains that seemed to spread throughout my body. The anesthesia had left me in a fog, and the strong medications they'd sent me home with did little to cut through it. I didn't remember much from that disorienting day other than drifting in and out of restless dreams.

As the haze began to lift on the second day's morning, it brought with it a new torment - sharp, stabbing pains that gripped my chest with every slight movement. I'd never experienced anything like it; it felt as though someone was twisting my muscles in different directions. Just lying still did little to ease the agony. Anytime I tried to lift my arm or turn in bed, fresh waves of pain would wash over me.

The medications helped remove the edge but did little to overcome the soreness. I was used to relying on pills just to get through each hour. My sleep schedule grew unpredictable as well, as I'd drift in and out of consciousness at all hours of the day and night. My sister, Joyceling, came to check on me and help with basic tasks like showering, which I could barely manage independently.

Yet the worst suffering was looking in the mirror those first few days. Where my breasts had been was now just a hollowed, scarred reminder of what I'd lost. I feared raising my eyes to my reflection, feeling a sense of trauma and loss at how radically my body had changed. Intellectually, I knew it was for the best in the long run, but emotionally it was devasting. It was the lowest point of my recovery so far, facing what this struggle had done to my sense of self and femininity. The physical pain faded in comparison to that inner distress.

The weeks after my surgery were a battle against me as I fluctuated between wanting a positive outlook and being dragged down by painful thoughts. Rationally, I knew this struggle was for the best in the long run, but emotionally, I struggled with feelings of loss over what had been taken from my body.

Though my husband took care of me on a daily basis and nurtured me with his pumpkin soup and encouraging words, my daughters gave all their smiles and company in the afternoons, and my parents visited faithfully each day, more often than not. I was only indistinctly aware of their presence through a fog of medication. My friends also tried to reach out, but their calls and texts would find me drifting in and out of restless sleep. On rare occasions, I was clear-headed and lacked the energy or will to respond properly.

I spent nearly all my time restricted to bed, drifting between fitful dozes. My children did their best to cheer me with visits after school, and for their sake, I'd try to shake myself and act like my normal, cheerful self. But the truth was I was depressed, wanting only to escape into unconsciousness through sleep or painkillers. My husband gently encouraged me to walk around the house, as the doctor had advised, but most days, even that seemed overwhelming.

I started to resent my decision, questioning if this alteration to my body had truly been worth it, even as logic said it was the right choice. My husband took on the burden of responsibilities, caring for me and our family with patience and compassion.

Yet despite his support, I felt lost in a dark place, unable to comprehend what was happening both physically and mentally in those early weeks. It was a constant push and pull between hope for healing and the despair of loss. The weeks blurred together as my struggle continued. I fought a constant battle within myself, trying to maintain optimism even as depressive thoughts drained what little energy I had. My body worked to heal while my mind tortured me further.

One morning in mid-October, I received a call that gave me a glimmer of light. It was my breast surgeon calling to deliver the results of the sentinel lymph node biopsy. To my immense relief, she informed me the cancer had not spread. I knew I would not need chemotherapy or medication. At that moment, all the fear and darkness lifted. I gathered the strength to publicly share the good news through social media. After that, my weekly follow-ups with my plastic surgeon began. The goal was to slowly expand the temporary implants over time through saline injections. But each appointment brought fresh pain that my depressed state made so much harder to face. Leaving my bed took more willpower than I had most days.

The prospect of those biweekly procedures stretching into the fall and winter seemed overwhelming. Yet my surgeon's call proved there was reason for hope, if only I could find the resilience to keep going one step at a time.

Finding the resilience took all my energy, but having my family lifting my spirits was essential in this journey.

As Halloween approached, my sisters Jaqui and Caty were adamant that we dress up as the Sanderson sisters from Hocus Pocus, a film we had loved since childhood. We always wanted to dress like the Sanderson sisters. However, I worried I wouldn't have the energy to dress up, but my sisters assured me they would help in any way needed. They lovingly assisted me, and I could have wept with gratitude. We even recreated lines from the movies, and it was indeed an unforgettable experience.

The young girl in me was extremely happy as my sisters, and I felt as if we were little again. For a moment, the laughs and smiles shared filled me with inexplicable strength more than any medicine ever could.

This chapter closes as my physical recovery transitions into the next phase. Though the road remains long, that single ray of light gave me cause to believe brighter days may yet lie ahead.

Chapter 6: Warrior Within - Discovering Strength Amidst Struggle

After facing those difficult experiences, I started focusing more on learning how to accept myself as I was. I was going through a process of coming to terms with the changes and scars on my body after surgery. At first, it was challenging to adjust to my new me. Over time, though, I began appreciating how far I'd come. I found myself looking at my scars less critically and more with gratitude. I realized just how lucky I am to be alive and still able to enjoy time with my family.

The appreciation for small blessings really started to sink in. Instead of dwelling on how things used to be, I focused on all the good things still in my life, like being here for my kids and husband. Those texts, cards, calls, and visits of support meant so much, reminding me of others' care during a tough period. I'm at a place now where I can reflect on my journey with humility rather than frustration. That process of shifting perspective continued for me. While there were certainly still low points where sadness would creep in, I was making strides to lift myself up again each time.

The first month after my procedure was truly difficult; the recovery was long and painful while still dealing with weekly follow-up appointments. Each time I went in to gradually fill my expanders, it proved to be extremely uncomfortable.

The expanders made me acutely aware of how unnatural my body still felt. For those first couple of months, it was especially like having two foreign objects continuously held inside me. The expanders didn't move or feel like natural tissue. Their rigid presence made regular activities like lying down or getting dressed quite awkward. The tightness and pressure were a constant reminder that my body wasn't quite my own yet. Despite the rough patches, I tried focusing on positive steps. Not needing chemotherapy or long-term medication gave me so much relief. As someone still learning to accept her "new normal," small victories took on a greater meaning. My support system also played a big role in boosting my spirit whenever my strength began to fade.

Each passing week brought gradual yet meaningful improvement in both my physical and mental well-being. There were certainly still struggles during my recovery process. Emotions like depression, anxiety, and lowered self-esteem each took their toll on me at various points.

However, it was comforting to know that the process had to end at some point. But at the moment, dealing with new pains, limitations, and emotions each week took a lot of mental adjustment. While the expanders came with discomfort, they did allow me to regain a sense of femininity through their shaping effects. I have some form of fullness in my chest again. Although artificial, they helped boost my confidence each time I got dressed. It kept reminding me of my eventual goal of looking whole once more.

My love-hate feelings towards the expanders started to take form. On one hand, they gave me back a silhouette that I sorely missed during those first few months. But their very presence also symbolized all the difficulties that were yet to come. Each filling meant that the finishing line was still far away while progress was being made. It was a trade-off to simultaneously find meaning in the positives and negatives.

Over time, those ups helped counterbalance the inevitable downs that came with the territory of healing. Focusing on small victories like expanding cups or their looseness kept hopes afloat for the final results. The light at the end of the proverbial tunnel grew bit by bit with each filling.

The uncomfortable feeling of expanders and their functionality, to me, made their necessity start to feel worthwhile. Those final months of recovery flew by in a blur of fillings, painkillers, depression, and rest. By the time late November rolled around, I had reached my limit. The expanders had done their job structurally, but mentally, I was extremely worn down.

When I met with my doctor for that last scheduled expansion before my intended return to work in early December, I knew that I needed to speak up. I explained to him how little energy I had, finding it a struggle just to care for basic needs. Just the idea of jumping back into a full-time work schedule left me feeling overwhelmed. My doctor kindly listened to my concerns without judgment. He understood that healing was about more than just physical milestones; the emotional and mental components were just as crucial. We agreed to postpone my return date slightly longer. That would allow me more time to regain my strength.

It was a relief to have that candid discussion. Slowing down, I permitted myself to fully recuperate without unnecessary pressure. I learned the important lesson that small delays in big plans can make all the difference when recovery isn't just about checking boxes but truly finding wholeness again on all levels. I knew that one more month of rest would serve me far better in the long run.

As I mentioned, part of my job involves leading a team supporting over 200 retail locations. December is our peak season, when stores are busiest. The idea of jumping back to full responsibility in that environment triggered major anxiety, given how limited my energy still was. Basic daily tasks like eating with family or maintaining hygiene felt extremely taxing. I could barely manage routine self-care from home. So, trying to also provide guidance and problem-solving for others while on my own journey to recovery seemed a far-fetched idea. My job demands high engagement, organization, and timely decision-making. At that stage of recovery, I questioned if I was realistically up for such demands, both physically and mentally.

I didn't want to shortchange my work or push myself too far before fully healing. Risking another setback didn't seem prudent either. I began experiencing panic attacks in anticipation of the upcoming busy season at work in December. This time of year requires providing constant support and handling escalations and emergencies. It involves long work hours when I must juggle numerous tasks simultaneously. While I barely managed to complete my regular duties, assuming an even heavier workload was too much for me. Just thinking about having to take on more responsibilities on top of an already full plate was overwhelming. I struggled with doing even the minimum required for my role. The pressure of

December and what it demands was really getting to me mentally.

I informed at work that I could not foresee being well enough in just a week to get in my car, bring my laptop, a large purse, and everything else I need, and successfully perform all my job duties during our busiest time of year. I couldn't understand how my mental and physical state could possibly be up to the challenges that time of year would bring. Everyone recovers at different rates, and I knew I was not ready. I told them that for my job responsibilities starting again on December 6th, it might realistically take me closer to three months to feel ready. In hindsight, the extra time off work helped me recover mostly. It reduced a lot of anxiety and stress I was under.

During that month, it hit me that I could not keep merely getting by and doing the bare minimum daily. I needed to start working on improving my condition and building up my abilities again if I wanted to resume my normal activities and duties.

Although things could not go back exactly how they had been before due to the changes, I realized that I needed to establish a new normal routine for myself, and I was still not fully prepared physically or mentally to handle my job responsibilities again. I understood that I could no longer continue what I had been doing, as it wasn't getting me anywhere closer to my new normal and independence once more. A change in approach was clearly needed. However, that period also served as a major wake-up call. I realized how depressed I had become by just barely managing to get through each day doing the bare minimum. That was simply not sustainable and not truly representative of who I am. It made me understand that I needed to shift my perspective and work on establishing a new normal routine for myself moving forward. Staying in that depressed mindset was getting me nowhere.

So, during that month before my new return date, I made the important decision to finally seek out therapy. I hadn't done so before then, but speaking with a professional counselor was invaluable. It helped me process what I had been through and start developing strategies to improve my mental and physical well-being. I also began reconnecting with online support groups for women who have dealt with similar health issues. I joined different Facebook support groups that have also battled breast cancer. That's where I found out that breast cancer survivors refer to each other as Pink sisters. I participated in chats, answered questions to women just being diagnosed, posted questions, and just being around others who truly understood what I was experiencing made a huge difference.

Through therapy and extensive self-help reading, I began focusing on improving my daily routine. Baby steps like getting out of bed, taking a shower, and getting dressed felt like victories.

Gentle arm exercises were added to what I could manage each day. This was a big shift from the prior month, where I had mainly just laid in bed doing the bare minimum to attend doctor appointments. I knew that I only had this one month before my return to work date, so my recovery became my main priority. While pushing myself provided motivation, it also came with lingering work-related anxiety. After getting used to doing so little, the uncertainty of whether I could truly handle my job responsibilities again was daunting. But I was always aware that avoiding that challenge would not help my situation either.

Each small accomplishment, such as making it through a full day without returning to bed, helped boost my confidence little by little. Checking in regularly with my support network and counselor kept me accountable and provided encouragement during setbacks.

Slowly but surely, I started to feel like my old self again, or at least a functional version of my new normal self. While nerve-wracking, going back to my daily work life seemed like a more realistic goal by the time the first week of January arrived. I went through a phase where I wasn't very active or productive. At times, my mind struggled to comprehend how I would get there; however, each day, my thoughts were focused on small improvements. I knew that if I improved just 1% each day, it would add up over time. So, each week, I would set small goals to work on. An early goal was simply getting out of bed and spending most of my time on the couch or walking around my living room instead of resting in bed. Even small movements left me feeling tired as my body worked to recover. I shifted my focus to tiny wins that helped me feel a sense of progress each day rather than feeling overwhelmed by how far I still had to go.

One goal was to spend more time in the living room than in my bedroom. Another was dressing in casual clothes rather than pajamas or having my husband help brush my hair and apply face cream. I kept a narrow focus on getting incrementally better each day rather than thinking about the larger challenges ahead. My daily improvements added up over time, even if they seemed minor individually. I was around two weeks away from planning to return to work when Christmas arrived. It was December, but the holidays were difficult for me that year. Normally, I would have been the one to buy presents, decorate the house, and kick off Christmas festivities right after Thanksgiving with shopping trips and other traditions. But that year, I didn't have the energy for any of that.

When Christmas was just around the corner, I began feeling anxious again.

The holidays were approaching, and internally, I didn't feel as recovered as I had hoped to be by that point. The anxiety began with wanting to enjoy Christmas fully with my family but realizing emotionally and mentally that I wasn't completely recharged yet. There was pressure I put on myself to be the same cheerful, upbeat person I had always been during this special time of year. Getting anxious showed me I still had lingering effects from what I had been through. The time for change was approaching, and I couldn't stop it from coming.

My husband handled our Christmas tree and basic decorations instead. While I was glad to see our home take on a festive look, it wasn't the same as my usual high level of involvement. I shared in the decorating in a limited way, but Christmas didn't have its usual feel without all our regular activities and rituals leading up to the day. It was definitely an adjustment to observe the changing season from the sidelines rather than actively participating as I normally would.

At the time, I thought it was okay to focus on getting better for the future. My kids weren't able to enjoy Christmas like usual, which caused feelings of guilt. I felt selfish for focusing on my own recovery instead of our normal holiday traditions. It was difficult dealing with depression and wondering why I felt this way. I questioned why I couldn't get better sooner. However, allowing myself to prioritize healing was important, too. My goal was to improve, even if that meant making sacrifices elsewhere initially. Things like our regular Christmas activities, which we enjoyed as a family, are now regrets. But I know that taking time for healing had to come first at that point. Given up on traditions and feelings of letting my kids down, it wasn't an easy decision.

One day, I woke up and noticed something odd about my face. My mom pointed it out to me after we took a family photo at Christmas. She asked what was going on with the way I looked. At first, I wasn't sure what she meant. But when I took a look at the picture myself, I saw that my smile was lopsided. One side of my mouth turned up higher than the other. My eye on that same side seemed droopy as well. It was strange because I hadn't noticed anything different about how I looked before that moment. But looking back at older photos, I could see subtle signs that something was shifting in my facial features over time. That Christmas picture was really the first time anyone had pointed it out directly to me, though.

Most days, I'd rush through a quick shower and throw on clean clothes, just focusing on basic hygiene. Naturally, I wasn't scrutinizing my face closely in the mirror anymore.

So, the subtle effects of progressing there went unnoticed by me at first. About two weeks before I was set to return to work, things took a scary turn. One morning, I woke up with partial paralysis on one side of my face. The loss of control was jarring and alarming. All of a sudden, I doubted if I was truly ready, mentally or physically, to return to the demands of my job. Even simple tasks, like driving myself, felt risky in that state. Everything felt like too much stress on my body and mind. It was possible all the pressure I was putting on myself to resume normal life was negatively impacting my recovery process, too. What I really wished for was more time.

On top of adjusting to expanders and the "new me," I also had to cope with losing control of half my face. The person looking back in the mirror hardly felt like herself anymore. And there was no hiding this change, unlike scars that could be covered by clothing.

I had been making progress in recent weeks, pushing myself to continue improving. But dealing with this latest setback erased so much of that hard-fought progress. When the paralysis hit, it truly felt like too much to bear. All I could think was, *"What else can possibly go wrong?"* At that point, I wasn't sure how much more I could genuinely handle. In a moment of desperation, I started searching feverishly online for anything that might provide relief or answers. That's when I came across information about facial yoga exercises. I was willing to try anything if it could potentially help. I downloaded some routine videos and diligently started the practice, doing the motions twice or even three times a day whenever I found the time. Within a few weeks, I began noticing improvements in my range of motion and control. The paralysis was slowly easing.

While my facial function didn't fully return to normal, it was a vast improvement over where I'd been. Even now, high-stress periods can sometimes make symptoms flare up slightly. But my only way to keep it under control is to stay consistent. I routinely performed yoga, which made a huge difference in my recovery process to the point that nobody at work noticed any lingering effects on my face when I finally returned to work. But privately, it added another source of worry as I adapted to many changes. Around that same time, my husband's chronic health issues also took a difficult turn. He has multiple sclerosis, and I think the combined stresses on our family have truly worn down his body. The week before I went back to work, he experienced an intense flare-up requiring an emergency hospital visit.

He was in excruciating pain, and I knew that I needed to drive him, even though I was still hesitant to drive myself after months away from it. Throughout everything, his own condition seemed to unconsciously sync up with or feed off my heightened stresses, and vice versa. When he went into that pain flare, I knew I had to act fast. I grabbed the car keys, saying, "I'm taking you right now." Driving was posing its own challenges, though. My arms still lacked full mobility after months of healing. I could only hold them close to my sides, secured in a place like they were tied there. That's how I steered and operated the vehicle—very slowly and carefully.

Understandably, other drivers grew impatient with my cautious speed. But I hadn't driven for so long; I was still healing, so I feared jeopardizing our safety. Navigating the familiar 10-minute route to the hospital felt unknown. Once we reached there, the medical staff explained that he needed to stay overnight for treatment and monitoring. Something about arthritis exacerbating in his spine caused immense suffering. It pained me to leave him like that when he'd done so much to support me through my own recovery.

His hospitalization right before I returned to my job just amplified the stress. At that point, it truly felt like event after event was piling up to challenge my mental fortitude. But looking back, I'm grateful my state of mind had regained some strength by then. It allowed me to manage an emergency situation level-headedly and focus on his care. Taking charge during a crisis like that gave me confidence that I was continuing to heal.

While the facial effects I faced likely seemed minor to outsiders, those small changes were still noticeable within my circle. It wasn't a huge transformation, but as the one living through it, I could detect where things hadn't fully returned to baseline.

When those events cascaded in rapid succession, all I could feel was, *"This is terrible."* The exhaustion wanted to take over. But something within pushed back, saying this situation demands strength—for my husband's care and our family's well-being too. So, a sense of resolution grew. I told myself I would rise to meet what was ahead by dedicating focused time to self-care. More practice with facial yoga videos and mindfulness became daily commitments. I think heading back to work was partially a way to start returning to my normal routine. At the time, getting out of bed and focusing on my recovery was a full-time job in itself. Driving again wasn't the best idea since I wasn't feeling like myself yet, and having to take my husband to the hospital unexpectedly made an already difficult situation feel much worse.

I don't think I would have felt ready to drive so soon—maybe not for another week, at least. The experience really made me more aware of what my body had been through. Not only was I still dealing with physical symptoms, but now there was the emotional challenge of coming to terms with the changes in my appearance. It was really hard to come to terms with the physical changes, especially since my face didn't look like what I remembered. Everything seemed droopy and unfamiliar. But now, when I think about this time of my life, I can see maybe all that happened for a reason. The recovery period made me embrace the changes in my appearance.

At least, that's how I try to frame it—focusing on the bright side and the positive things that came out of those situations.

I think the most important element connected to bringing positivity in you is the people you are with. If we surround ourselves with uplifting people and look inward, we can overcome anything. I felt it the most when things were dark; creative hobbies, self-reflection, and spiritual activities helped guide my way. I learned to appreciate small things that matter to us more than we think they do. My family and friends, the community group, the way they didn't let me succumb to depression, and the unconditional love from my husband and daughters were truly a blessing.

Healing is not a straight line; it is a very rocky path with a lot of lows and highs. Leaving you with feelings of great accomplishment and failures.

My dear breasties! One step at a time.

Chapter 7: Embracing Scars - A Journey of Body and Soul

After three months of not showing up at work, it was time to go back to my duties. I remember a peculiar feeling of nervousness spreading through my body like waves. I was mentally preparing myself to get back to my old life, where I used to work effortlessly. It had been a roller coaster for me and my family. Although the period of three months isn't such a long time, it did feel like it lasted longer than we thought it would. I believe time gets slower when we are not feeling our best.

In January, I went back to work. I remember the pain I felt with each bump on the road while driving to work and how I had to drive at the lowest speed to avoid any further pain. The feeling of getting back to work and meeting people there was filled with uneasiness as if it was my first day at work. I also doubted my ability to perform my responsibilities and manage a hundred stores like I used to. As a result, I could feel the pressure building up inside of me.

There was a time when I didn't want to get out of bed at all. I was depressed and huddled up on my bed, refusing to face the world. It was tough to get used to the new normal. My body was reacting to the trauma by showing visible signs of stress. And the idea of taking charge of my team like I used to put me under constant pressure. I knew these were the same tasks I had handled before, and even if a situation got a little out of control, I could always take care of them. However, this time, my mind was running through self-doubt.

What if I couldn't do my work efficiently? What if I have to re-learn everything? At this point, all I needed was assurance and support. My family and my team were quite supportive and understanding of my situation. It was my mind that was going over all places, and what I needed was self-assurance from myself.

Even with everything going on, I needed to know I could do it all over again. Oftentimes, it is our overthinking that gets us, and we feel helpless to suppress the surge of unmotivating thoughts. One thing I recognized was that I needed some motivation.

When I resumed my work, I began listening to motivational videos, audible books, and podcasts on my way to work. The struggle of putting myself together as the individual I used to be wasn't a linear path. There was a palpable realization of not feeling like myself again. It was nothing less than a struggle. It was like fighting against me in a way that a part of me wanted to almost give up because starting over is too much work. I found myself wondering if I had to rebuild my entire life and start from scratch because I felt so disconnected from who I used to be. Others might not be able to see my bodily changes, but I would inevitably look at the scars that reminded me of my pain every day. It was a challenge for me to begin to pick up my life where I had left it. All I needed was to figure out that I was still capable of doing everything I did pre-surgery.

To be honest, it was terrifying. Just walking the familiar path filled me with anxiety. Thankfully, my support system not only stood by me but also understood what I was going through. Their presence gave me the courage to return to work., I pushed through my mental and physical struggles and got back to my job.

Indeed, the people you have in your life make and break your confidence. Even when I doubted my capabilities, they didn't. It was their help and assurance that I took charge of projects and began managing the task I was assigned, which later turned out to be a positive change. I realized that I was no longer overthinking or revisiting what the past few months had been for me at work. It brought a positive change in me. I stayed busy, which kept my mind occupied despite feeling scared to go back initially; it aided my mental well-being.

It was a phase that showed me I'm capable of overcoming any situation and rebuilding my life, regardless of what I've been through. There is always a way out, even when the chances are slim. There is always something or someone out there who could be of help to you. I was fortunate to have supportive colleagues at work. Getting back into my routine, staying busy, and even starting coaching volleyball with my sister Jaqui in March all contributed to this realization.

As days went by, the time came to arrange my second surgery. Around mid-February, I reminded my boss about it. Even before returning to work, I had informed him about the scheduled surgery in March. Upon my return, I promptly reiterated this and informed him that another surgery was necessary for the reconstruction work. The exact date fell between March and April, and once I had it, I communicated it to my workplace.

I was so relieved that I didn't have to take FMLA or sick time off work for my surgery. My job let me take a week of vacation and work from home for another, which helped ease my mind. But as the date of March 16th got closer, all the fears came flooding back. Even though the doctors said this operation would be much quicker and less painful than before, I still felt so worried and scared. Hearing it would only take a week to start feeling better didn't make me less afraid. I was afraid of that white room and everything it meant. Just going to pre-surgery appointments brought back horrible memories and made my stomach churn with fear. I think what I went through gave me PTSD because any time I thought about surgery, I got overwhelmed with panic and anxiety. The closer it got, the more terrified I felt. The white walls, the bright lighting, and the atmosphere of a hospital passing through hallways all came flushing back into my mind.

I knew deep down this reconstruction was important for my health and healing.

But in those weeks before, it was a daily struggle just to function through all the emotions. I felt so alone in my fears and didn't know if I could face going under the knife again. I just wanted it over but dreaded what was to come.

As the surgery date grew closer, I felt more and more afraid. I knew I had to get everything in order first, but it was so stressful. At work, I made sure all my tasks were handed off properly for the week I'd be gone. At home, too, I constantly check that everything is taken care of.

So many worries filled my head during that tense time. Even though the doctors said this wouldn't be as bad, it didn't stop the fears flooding in after all I'd already suffered. Going through something so traumatic before left deep scars that therapy couldn't fully heal.

All the old panic and terror resurfaced, leaving me an anxious wreck. No amount of reassurance could shake the dark thoughts swirling in my mind. Surgery day arrived all too soon, with nothing but dread dragging my weary body to the pre-op room. It was still so early, and I felt utterly alone despite my surgeon's calm presence.

This time, at least, it was just my plastic surgeon doing the reconstructive work instead of multiple doctors performing different procedures. But meeting with him to finalize details only brought on more worries as the reality set in. I didn't know how I'd find the courage to face those operating doors again after last time's horrors. All I felt was fear of the unknown pain ahead.

My surgeon and I had previously discussed fat grafting as an option for my breast reconstruction procedure. Fat grafting involves using one's own liposuctioned fat deposits to add natural-looking fullness and projection to the breasts. Rather than solely relying on implants, which can give an artificially hollow appearance, fat grafting was proposed to give a softer, more cohesive shape.

On the day of surgery, March 16th, my plastic surgeon met with me again in the pre-op room to finalize details. We gently reviewed the process, where small amounts of fat would be harvested using liposuction from agreed-upon donor sites like my stomach or thighs. This autologous fat would then be carefully grafted above the breast tissue in gradual layers for an organically rounded profile. While implants could provide desirable volume alone, it was hoped fat grafting's living fat cells would take and integrate naturally. This blended approach aimed to realistically mimic the look and feel of healthy breast tissue with no obvious demarcation between augmentation and natural structures.

Ultimately, the goal was a balanced, symmetrical result, bringing reconstruction and comfort while respecting my personal goals for a discreet yet confident appearance.

When the day of surgery arrived, my anxiety was skyrocketing. As the nurses prepared to take me to the operating room, I had a full-blown panic attack, just like last time. I was overwhelmed with flashbacks to my previous surgery and terrified of the unknown. I hugged my husband before leaving for my surgery. He had been a great emotional support in these times of need when I was surrounded by stress and whatnot. Panic set in when I woke up in the room I was shifted to. I was shocked by how swollen and large my breasts appeared.

The nurses and even my doctor reassured me the size was simply due to swelling, but I worried it looked unnatural. Their assurances did little to ease my anxiety at that moment. I wasn't happy with the appearance of my chest.

In the following days, my healing progressed much faster than expected. Mobility returned quickly, and the pain proved easier to manage in hindsight. I knew I had to be patient with the results, and to my relief, the swelling went down, and my breasts appeared in a natural shape and size, returning a sense of comfort. After a week of recovery, I was able to start working from home remotely, lifting my spirits with the routine. Working from home was not a hurdle for me, given that the first surgery didn't have a good impact on me. The first surgery was such an ordeal, both physically and emotionally draining. But having the reconstruction done has made all the difference. Recovery was so much easier this time around.

Not only does my body feel less pain, but my spirit feels lighter. Having breasts that look natural again has given me back a sense of myself as a woman. My clothes fit comfortably once more, and I carry myself with greater confidence each day.

This time, it was much easier for my body to start feeling better. I could move around without as much pain. But healing my mind has helped, too. Every small step of getting better takes me farther from the scary, hard times before. Putting in the implants meant finishing the last part of my surgery journey. Now that it's over, I'm hoping for better days ahead. Those painful memories don't drag me down like they used to. I took back my health and myself through all of this. Even though the scars will stay with me, I will learn to love them one day, as they have taught me the valuable lesson of becoming stronger even when I don't feel like getting up from my comfort zone. Each morning is now a chance for me to feel good again and be grateful for the health God has blessed me with.

With my experience in the past, I accepted what my body had been through as a part of the journey we call life. Enduring the pain and rising above it all is an accomplishment for anyone where you tell yourself, *"You did it even when you thought you couldn't."*

Now that I am moving forward, I am certain that nothing could stop me. My mind and my body are powerful and capable of healing.

Chapter 8: Radiant Support - Love and Solidarity in the Battle

By the third week following my surgery, it was finally time to resume work duties. Surprisingly, the transition back wasn't as excruciating as I had thought it would be, unlike my previous experience post-surgery. A sense of relief washed over me, knowing that I wouldn't have to endure the same level of discomfort while carrying out even the simplest tasks. It turned out to be a much smoother process than I had feared, and honestly, that was an immense relief.

As my body gradually healed from the ordeal, I felt ready to step back into the world. This time, there was a noticeable change in my outlook. I found a brand new confidence in my body. Something I had been lacking for the past few months. It wasn't that I despised my body or its appearance, but rather, it was the scars that left me feeling self-conscious about my journey. After my reconstructive surgery, I experienced a significant shift within myself. I began to feel comfortable in my own skin again, as if a spark had reignited within me. The sense of insecurity I once carried started to fade away. Clothes fit me better; gradually, everything seemed to fall into place. This sensation was deeply personal and difficult to put into words. While I couldn't say I loved my healing body outright, I did learn the importance of accepting myself just as I am.

Even during my lowest moments, I realized the need to show myself kindness and care. After all, we're all aging, and our bodies undergo various transformations along the way. Embracing each stage of this journey became essential to me. Life taught me a lesson of self-acceptance again, but this time, it meant so much more to me. This body of ours is a vessel that carries us through life's ups and downs. When my confidence was restored, there was a boast of assurance. This transformation whispered to me the power I had within me. Life indeed tests us to bring out our capabilities we wouldn't know otherwise. I knew I was stronger than the challenges in my way. My post-surgery made me see my potential to handle any hurdle I encounter.

There was a sense of getting back to my old self. The way I used to be. I was grateful, happy, and excited to regain my life. I felt like I was back in the world as a winner.

One thing I certainly and strongly felt was a change in my perspective. How I used to see things had clearly changed and changed for good. Everything, even with its scant significance, has a meaning in life. We take things for granted because we fail to see beyond our worries and problems and miss our happy moments. In the year 2022, everything was transformed for me. I was able to see the meaning behind every small thing. Perhaps a newer way of looking at things that surround me, and I no longer want to miss the opportunity to enjoy life's beautiful moments, for they are short-lived. Every little thing felt like it mattered.

In April, I turned 41, just after my surgery. It was unlike any other birthday. It felt like a celebration of life, being grateful for another year in this world with my loved ones. Waking up that day felt incredible. I was filled with gratitude, which made me feel amazing. Turning 41 had a deeper meaning after everything I went through. All I wanted was to be surrounded by my family, so we went to a Peruvian restaurant in the D.C. area and enjoyed each other's company. It was simple but beautiful, and that birthday meant a lot to me. That year, I was in a mindset of not putting off things I always wanted to do because life is unpredictable. I started journaling again, something I loved but had neglected. I also focused on my love for plants, making sure my home was filled with them. Having plenty of plants around brings me so much joy and positive energy. It's like having my own little green sanctuary.

I prioritized my love for reading and listening to books. It's my "me time," where I can escape into different worlds and scenarios. During the routine of being a mom and working, I had stopped making time for this hobby, but I realized how much I missed it. So, I made it a priority to read and listen to books again. I even got an Audible membership to make it easier to access a variety of titles.

I made a conscious effort to focus on things that truly make me happy and not waste time on anything else. Life is too short to ignore our passions and desires. This year, I vowed to cherish every moment and pursue the things that bring me joy and fulfillment. In essence, I kept myself busy and close with my family and friends. There was a lot of healing happening within me. And I knew that I was content with everything I was doing. Working and then home, I began to give my hundred percent, and I couldn't be more grateful that life gave me another chance to do all these things once again.

There was certainly a newfound sense of not taking things for granted and living life to the fullest. The following year, after I recovered from my surgery, my goal was to prioritize what meant the most to me—my children, my husband, my family, my friends, and what I love to do in my life.

That year, one of my main priorities was ensuring quality time with my girls. All too often in the past, I would come home tired from work and not give them my full attention, but I vowed things would be different. I wanted to make weekday evenings relaxing times where we could play games as a family and talk about our day.

I also had a strong urge to travel more and have memorable experiences. In April, I organized a family reunion in Tulum, Mexico, so my parents, mother-in-law, and sisters could reconnect during the summer. It was just what we all needed. In May, we traveled to Tampa to celebrate my youngest sister's graduation from medical school - a huge accomplishment. As someone who helped me through my own health issues, I was proud to be there for her.

June found us beachside in Tulum. The scenery was stunning, but what made it truly special was the joy of sharing that time with loved ones. Tulum has a special space in my heart. The cenotes, crystal waters, boho house, white sand, palm trees, Laguna Kaan Lumm, fresh mango, and blue skies are part of this mesmerized place's great memories. Right before the summer ended, just my immediate family took a weekend trip to one of the local beaches near our home. Listening to waves crashing, our feet touching the sand, and enjoying the sunsets is one of our favorite places to be.

Every experience that year reinforced how short life can be. I didn't want to look back with regrets, so I made an effort to seize opportunities while I could. Finances were carefully managed, but experiences with family took priority. It was the fulfillment I'd hoped to find by living each moment to the fullest.

The trips and time with loved ones rejuvenated me in a way I hadn't felt for years. As fall arrived and a new school year began, I was determined to carry that sense of renewed priorities and meaning into our daily lives. Our weeknights became focused on home-cooked dinners together, followed by games as a family. On weekends, simple pleasures like hiking, planting, biking, and baking replaced our former habit of constantly rushing from one activity to the next.

As the chill of winter set in, our travels shifted to more low-key excursions like coffee time or ice skating trips. On holidays, we hosted both sides of the extended family for meals and fun. Laughter filled our home in a way I'd nearly forgotten was possible.

Chapter 9: Milestones & Setbacks

The year 2022 filled me with gratitude for the opportunities knocking at my door. I found happiness in doing what had been on my wishlist for a long time. Seeing my family coming together even stronger than before was nothing but beautiful. I absolutely love it when our family is together under the same roof, backing and uplifting each other up.

I have always wanted to visit places with my family, like going back to my native country, Peru, and visiting Cusco and Machu Picchu, which are among the seven wonders of the world. It was a mystical presence as we laid our eyes on what unfolded before us. The green mountains, big rocks, alpacas, paths, blue sky, coca leaves, and charming views are instilled in my soul—a lifetime memory with my family, my parents, and my siblings. I was grateful that I could visit this place with the people who matter to me the most. Being with my whole family brought me lots of happiness, especially seeing my kids experience it all. I wanted my children to be familiar with my cultural background. The trip to Peru meant more to me than I realized. The places we visited were amazing, but being with loved ones in such a special spot is what I'll always treasure the most.

Our time in Peru created memories that I know my kids will look back on with joy. Even though they're young now, I hope they'll understand one day how important that trip was for our family and for learning about where we come from.

After my surgeries and what followed after, soon I was on my feet recovering from the stitches. Every day, I wake up and feel grateful for how far we have come in life. And how the involvement of my friends and family and their immense love for me made my journey to recovery possible. Though there were setbacks and I lacked the motivation to work forward, I let my challenges know that I could surpass them in all ways. I knew if life was testing me through my well-being, then I would become even stronger and more resilient.

For all those who are fighting a battle within themselves every day, believe in yourself and don't underestimate the power in you; instead, unleash it. Don't let negative thoughts and doubts win against you.

Chapter 10: Legacy of Love - Inspiring others

In search of better things in life, we often forget to prioritize our own well-being. There is no denying that life happens, and naturally, we get so busy that we barely make time for ourselves and barely notice changes in our bodies.

Breast cancer is the most common type of cancer among women. What I went through while battling cancer was tough and demanding. It left me thinking about so many things at once. My life, my goals, what I wanted for myself and my kids, everything.

My journey of battling against breast cancer was filled with many challenges. The withdrawal of blood through my nipple was the beginning of what I would not have imagined myself with before. And here I was, contemplating and stressing about *how to deal with it.* Life showed me a new way of seeing and perceiving things. It blew right into my face with a brand new test of health issues. Life never really readies you for anything. Even if it was foretold to me that at some point in my life, I'd be in a hospital room prepping for a bilateral mastectomy and then dealing with the aftermath of it, I would still have doubts about getting surgery. In times like these, I couldn't help but wonder if the cancer was even there or if it was just a temporary bump.

However, the unannounced appearance of it grabbed me like a giant hand from somewhere and put me in a dark place where I had to learn to get used to it. And followed the pain of surgery, the stitches, the removal of my womanhood. I felt incomplete; a part of me was missing. *Will I ever get to see myself again the way I used to?* A question I found establishing within my confinements, hammering me quite so often. Let me tell you, each moment I went through and each time I saw myself and my body getting back to normal was worth it. It took time, effort, and my whole resilient self, which had broken many times in the process. Nothing would have been possible without the support and help of the people around me. I think it took a whole village to get through this.

I am grateful for the life that brought me here. It is said that the bad things that teach us the good things in life. These bad things bring out our true capabilities we wouldn't have known otherwise. I couldn't tell if it was my resilience or the love and support of my family, friends, and community that made me strong.

All the pain I endured, the restless nights and days, now, when I look back, I see myself going through all of it like a pro. I haven't forgotten any of it. Whatever I am today is because of my courage, resilience, and love from my children, husband, family, and friends. Love heals wounds of deep, and eventually, I learned to love myself again. My new body, the change in me.

Anyone who is going through this journey of battling against cancer or other disease, I want you to know that your willpower is the strength of your body and soul. You must find it and believe in finding it. Life allows us to learn and grow; every day is a new page of your life story. Know that you have the power to write it. Your story might not always be how you want, but you can still change it how you like.

After my recovery, I think I will forever cherish every moment of my life – big or small. We often forget that in this world, we have only been here for some time. Be kind to one another and cherish every little thing that is as significant in life as your achievements. Prioritizing your well-being is just as crucial as prioritizing your family. If you cannot take good care of yourself, how would you take care of your loved ones?

Learn to be positive about things. Having an optimistic mindset makes many things easier in life. Our state of mind either makes us do things or mess everything up. This dark moment can be turned into a bright one with a changed perspective. Even when I failed to remain positive about my condition, my family gave me hope. They uplifted me in many ways, and I will forever be grateful for their presence. God has truly blessed me in my tough times.

Dear fellow fighters, always remember that cancer is not just a mere battle we fight. It is way beyond that. Many people's efforts include doctors, nurses, staff, family, friends, and the community. I would like to thank everyone who took the time to read my story and be a part of this journey. My goal is to raise awareness about breast cancer as much as I can. No woman should be robbed of her womanhood through breast cancer. I hope that in the upcoming years, my story and my work to raise awareness will help woman deeply understand the importance of prioritizing their health.

Let the women you love and the women in your life know the importance of it and guide them if you do find someone with related symptoms. It is never wrong to get checked.

Be part of raising breast cancer awareness; be the change this world needs!